BEYOND AUTOIMMUNE DISEASE

A Holistic Approach to Reclaim Your Health

Blair O Joel

Copyright © 2024 by **Blair O Joel**

All rights reserved. No part of this book may be reproduced or transmitted in any form or by any means, electronic or mechanical, including photocopying, recording, or by any information storage and retrieval system, without permission in writing from the author.

TABLE OF CONTENT

BEYOND AUTOIMMUNE DISEASE 1

INTRODUCTION 7

    Understanding the Enemy Within 7

    Common Autoimmune Conditions... 12

    The Immune System and Its Role 15

    How Autoimmune Diseases Develop... 18

THE IMPACT OF AUTOIMMUNE DISEASES 21

    Physical and Emotional Symptoms 21

    Quality of Life and Daily Challenges... 22

    Impact on Relationships and Family 23

    Economic and Social Consequences 25

TRADITIONAL MEDICAL APPROACHES 29

    Medications and Their Side Effects.. 29

    Surgery and Its Risks.. 31

    The Limitations of Conventional Treatments.................................. 33

THE SEARCH FOR CURES 35

    Current Research and Advancements... 35

    Emerging Therapies and Their Potential 37

    The Challenges in Developing Effective Treatments 38

LIFESTYLE AND ENVIRONMENTAL FACTORS 41

    The Role of Diet and Nutrition 41

    Stress Management and Relaxation Techniques 43

    Exercise and Physical Activity 45

    Environmental Toxins and Their Impact 46

ACUPUNCTURE AND ACUPRESSURE 49

    Acupuncture and Acupressure 49

    Common Herbal Remedies: 51

    Chiropractic Care and Massage Therapy 52

    Mindfulness and Meditation 54

HOLISTIC APPROACHES TO HEALING 57

    The Mind-Body Connection 57

    Emotional and Spiritual Well-Being 58

    Personalized Healing Plans 60

PERSONAL NARRATIVES 63

    Inspiring Stories of Individuals Overcoming Autoimmune Challenges 63

    Lessons Learned and Strategies for Coping 65

HOPE FOR THE FUTURE 67

    The Power of Advocacy and Awareness 67

    Embracing a Positive Outlook 68

    The Potential for a Brighter Future 69

PERSONAL NOTES 71

INTRODUCTION

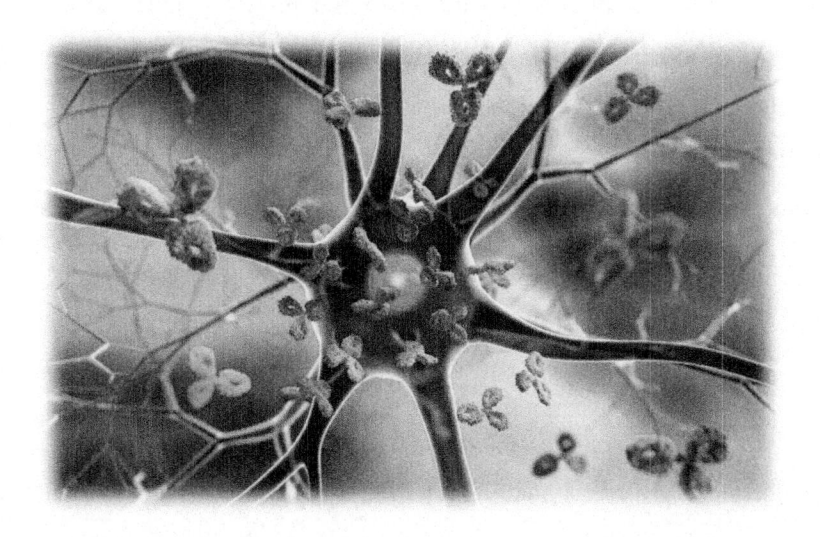

Understanding the Enemy Within

Autoimmune diseases, once considered rare, are now recognized as a growing public health concern. They affect millions of people worldwide, causing a wide range of symptoms and varying degrees of severity. This chapter delves into the fundamental aspects of autoimmune diseases, providing a clear understanding of what they are, how they develop, and the challenges they pose.

What is an Autoimmune Disease?

An autoimmune disease occurs when the body's immune system, designed to protect against invaders like bacteria and viruses, mistakenly attacks its own tissues. This misdirected assault can lead to inflammation, tissue damage, and a host of symptoms. Unlike infectious diseases caused by external pathogens, autoimmune diseases are internal battles fought within the body.

The Immune System: A Brief Overview

To comprehend autoimmune diseases, it is essential to have a basic understanding of the immune system. This intricate network of cells, tissues, and organs acts as the body's defense mechanism. It comprises two primary components:

- Innate Immunity: This is the first line of defense, providing a rapid but general response to threats. It includes physical barriers like skin and mucous membranes, as well as cells like neutrophils and macrophages that engulf and destroy invaders.
- Adaptive Immunity: This is a more targeted and slower response that develops over time. It involves lymphocytes, including T cells and B cells, which recognize and attack specific antigens (foreign substances).

The Breakdown: How Autoimmune Diseases Develop

The exact causes of autoimmune diseases remain a subject of ongoing research, but several factors are believed to contribute to their development:

- Genetic Predisposition: Certain genes may make individuals more susceptible to autoimmune diseases. These genes can influence the immune system's function and regulation.
- Environmental Triggers: Exposure to environmental factors, such as infections, toxins, or stress, can trigger an autoimmune response in genetically predisposed individuals.
- Hormonal Factors: Hormones can play a role in the development of autoimmune diseases. For example, autoimmune thyroid diseases are more common in women, likely due to hormonal fluctuations.
- Immune System Dysregulation: In autoimmune diseases, the immune system becomes dysregulated, losing its ability to distinguish between self and non-self. This can lead to the attack of healthy tissues.

Common Autoimmune Diseases

Autoimmune diseases can affect virtually any part of the body. Some of the most common conditions include:

- Rheumatoid Arthritis: A chronic inflammatory disease that affects the joints, causing pain, swelling, and stiffness.
- Multiple Sclerosis (MS): A neurological disease that damages the myelin sheath surrounding nerve fibers, leading to a variety of symptoms, including weakness, numbness, and vision problems.
- Type 1 Diabetes: An autoimmune condition that destroys insulin-producing cells in the pancreas, resulting in high blood sugar levels.
- Systemic Lupus Erythematosus (SLE): A systemic autoimmune disease that can affect multiple organs, causing symptoms like fatigue, joint pain, and skin rashes.
- Psoriasis: A chronic skin condition characterized by patches of thick, red, scaly skin.
- Crohn's Disease and Ulcerative Colitis: Inflammatory bowel diseases that affect the digestive tract, causing symptoms like abdominal pain, diarrhea, and weight loss.
- Celiac Disease: An autoimmune condition triggered by the consumption of gluten, a protein found in wheat, barley, and rye.

The Growing Burden of Autoimmune Diseases

The prevalence of autoimmune diseases has been increasing in recent years. This can be attributed to several factors, including:

- Improved Diagnosis: Advances in medical technology and diagnostic techniques have led to a more accurate identification of autoimmune diseases.
- Environmental Changes: Factors such as pollution, exposure to chemicals, and changes in lifestyle may contribute to the development of autoimmune diseases.
- Aging Population: As the global population ages, the incidence of autoimmune diseases is expected to rise, as many of these conditions are more common in older adults.

Challenges and Outlook

Despite significant progress in understanding and treating autoimmune diseases, many challenges remain. These include:

- Lack of Cures: Most autoimmune diseases do not have a cure, and treatment often focuses on managing symptoms and preventing complications.
- Variability in Symptoms: Autoimmune diseases can present with a wide range of symptoms, making diagnosis and treatment complex.
- Coexisting Conditions: Many individuals with autoimmune diseases also have other health conditions, which can complicate their management.

Common Autoimmune Conditions

Autoimmune diseases occur when the body's immune system mistakenly attacks its own tissues. There are hundreds of autoimmune conditions, each with its unique set of symptoms. Here are some of the most common ones:

Rheumatic Diseases

Rheumatoid Arthritis: A chronic inflammatory disease that affects the joints, causing pain, swelling, and stiffness.

- Lupus: A systemic autoimmune disease that can affect multiple organs, causing symptoms like fatigue, joint pain, and skin rashes.
- Scleroderma: A rare autoimmune disease that causes the skin and connective tissues to thicken and harden.

Gastrointestinal Diseases

- Crohn's Disease: An inflammatory bowel disease that can affect any part of the digestive tract, causing symptoms like abdominal pain, diarrhea, and weight loss.

- Ulcerative Colitis: Another inflammatory bowel disease that primarily affects the large intestine, causing symptoms like bloody diarrhea and abdominal cramps.
- Celiac Disease: An autoimmune condition triggered by the consumption of gluten, a protein found in wheat, barley, and rye.

Endocrine Diseases

- Type 1 Diabetes: An autoimmune disease that destroys insulin-producing cells in the pancreas, resulting in high blood sugar levels.
- Hashimoto's Thyroiditis: An autoimmune condition that attacks the thyroid gland, leading to hypothyroidism.
- Graves' Disease: An autoimmune condition that causes the thyroid gland to produce too much thyroid hormone.

Neurological Diseases

- Multiple Sclerosis (MS): A chronic autoimmune disease that affects the central nervous system, causing symptoms like fatigue, weakness, and vision problems.
- Myasthenia Gravis: An autoimmune disease that affects the muscles, causing weakness and fatigue.
- Skin Diseases
- Psoriasis: A chronic skin condition characterized by patches of thick, red, scaly skin.

- Atopic Dermatitis: A chronic skin condition that causes itchy, red, and inflamed skin.

Other Common Autoimmune Conditions
- ✓ Raynaud's Phenomenon: A condition that causes the fingers and toes to become numb and cold in response to cold temperatures or stress.
- ✓ Sjögren's Syndrome: A condition that affects the moisture-producing glands in the body, causing dry eyes and dry mouth.
- ✓ Pernicious Anemia: An autoimmune condition that interferes with the body's ability to absorb vitamin B12.

The Immune System and Its Role

The immune system is a complex network of cells, tissues, and organs that work together to protect the body from harmful invaders such as bacteria, viruses, fungi, and parasites. It is a vital component of the body's defense mechanism.

The Two Main Components of the Immune System

The immune system consists of two primary components:

- ✓ Innate Immunity: This is the first line of defense, providing a rapid but general response to threats. It includes physical barriers like skin and mucous membranes, as well as cells like neutrophils and macrophages that engulf and destroy invaders.
- ✓ Adaptive Immunity: This is a more targeted and slower response that develops over time. It involves lymphocytes, including T cells and B cells, which recognize and attack specific antigens (foreign substances).

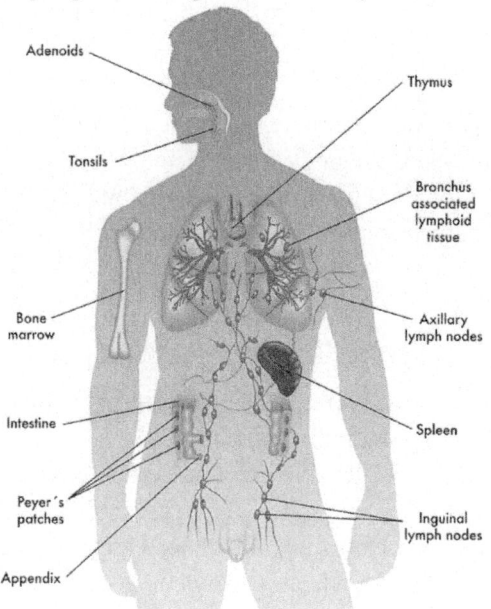

How the Immune System Works
- When a foreign invader enters the body, the immune system responds in a coordinated effort:
- Recognition: The immune system recognizes the invader as foreign and identifies its unique antigens.
- Activation: Specialized cells, such as macrophages and dendritic cells, present the antigens to T cells and B cells, activating them.
- Attack: T cells and B cells work together to eliminate the invader. T cells directly attack infected cells, while B cells produce antibodies that bind to the invader and mark it for destruction.
- Memory: The immune system retains memory of the invader, allowing it to respond more quickly and effectively if it encounters the same threat in the future.

The Importance of a Healthy Immune System

A healthy immune system is essential for maintaining good health. It protects the body from infections and diseases, and it helps to heal wounds and injuries. When the immune system is compromised, a person is more susceptible to illness.

Factors Affecting Immune Function
- Several factors can affect the function of the immune system, including:
- Age: The immune system weakens as people age, making older adults more susceptible to infections.
- Nutrition: A balanced diet with adequate nutrients is essential for a healthy immune system.
- Stress: Chronic stress can weaken the immune system.

- o Sleep: Lack of sleep can impair immune function.
- o Medications: Some medications, such as corticosteroids, can suppress the immune system.
- o Underlying medical conditions: Certain medical conditions, such as HIV/AIDS and autoimmune diseases, can weaken the immune system.

Maintaining a Healthy Immune System

To support a healthy immune system, it is important to:

- o Eat a balanced diet: Consume plenty of fruits, vegetables, whole grains, and lean protein.
- o Get enough sleep: Aim for 7-8 hours of sleep per night.
- o Manage stress: Practice stress-reduction techniques such as meditation, yoga, or deep breathing.
- o Exercise regularly: Regular physical activity can boost immune function.
- o Avoid excessive alcohol and tobacco: These substances can weaken the immune system.
- o Stay up-to-date on vaccinations: Vaccines can help protect against infectious diseases.

How Autoimmune Diseases Develop

The exact causes of autoimmune diseases remain a subject of ongoing research, but several factors are believed to contribute to their development:

Genetic Predisposition

- o Hereditary Factors: Certain genes may make individuals more susceptible to autoimmune diseases. These genes can influence the immune system's function and regulation.
- o Family History: People with a family history of autoimmune diseases are at a higher risk of developing them themselves.

Environmental Triggers

- o Infections: Exposure to certain viruses or bacteria can trigger an autoimmune response in susceptible individuals.
- o Toxins: Exposure to environmental toxins, such as pollutants and chemicals, can contribute to autoimmune diseases.
- o Stress: Chronic stress can disrupt the immune system's balance and increase the risk of autoimmune disorders.

Hormonal Factors

- o Hormone Imbalances: Hormonal fluctuations, particularly those related to puberty, pregnancy, and menopause, can influence the development of autoimmune diseases.

- Sex Differences: Some autoimmune diseases are more common in women than in men, suggesting a role for sex hormones.

Immune System Dysregulation
- Loss of Tolerance: In autoimmune diseases, the immune system loses its ability to distinguish between self and non-self. This can lead to the attack of healthy tissues.
- Genetic Abnormalities: Mutations in genes involved in immune system regulation can contribute to autoimmune diseases.

Epigenetics
Environmental Influences on Genes: Epigenetics refers to changes in gene expression that are not caused by changes in the DNA sequence. Environmental factors can influence epigenetic modifications, affecting the risk of autoimmune diseases.

The Complex Interaction of Factors
It is likely that a combination of these factors plays a role in the development of autoimmune diseases. The specific factors involved may vary depending on the individual and the type of autoimmune disease.

Ongoing Research

Scientists continue to investigate the underlying causes of autoimmune diseases in order to develop more effective treatments and prevention strategies. By understanding the complex interplay of genetic, environmental, and immunological factors, researchers hope to shed light on the development of these conditions.

THE IMPACT OF AUTOIMMUNE DISEASES

Physical and Emotional Symptoms

Autoimmune diseases can have a significant impact on both physical and emotional well-being. The specific symptoms vary depending on the type of autoimmune disease, but some common physical symptoms include:

- **Fatigue:** Feeling tired and exhausted, even after getting enough sleep
- **Pain:** Aching joints, muscles, or other parts of the body
- **Swelling:** Joint swelling or swelling in other areas of the body
- **Digestive problems:** Diarrhea, constipation, or abdominal pain
- **Skin problems:** Rashes, itching, or hair loss
- **Fever:** A higher than normal body temperature

In addition to physical symptoms, autoimmune diseases can also have a significant impact on emotional well-being. Some common emotional symptoms include:

- **Depression:** Feelings of sadness, hopelessness, or worthlessness
- **Anxiety:** Feelings of worry, fear, or nervousness

- **Stress:** Feeling overwhelmed or unable to cope
- **Frustration:** Feeling irritated or annoyed
- **Isolation:** Feeling alone or disconnected from others

Quality of Life and Daily Challenges

- Autoimmune diseases can significantly affect quality of life and daily activities. People with autoimmune diseases may face challenges such as:
- **Limited mobility:** Difficulty walking, standing, or sitting for extended periods
- **Difficulty performing daily tasks:** Trouble getting dressed, bathing, or preparing meals
- **Social isolation:** Feeling isolated from friends and family due to symptoms or limitations
- **Financial strain:** High medical costs and lost income can be financially burdensome
- **Difficulty maintaining a healthy lifestyle:** Challenges with diet, exercise, and sleep

Impact on Relationships and Family

Autoimmune diseases can have a profound impact on relationships and family dynamics. The physical and emotional symptoms of these conditions can strain relationships with loved ones, leading to feelings of frustration, resentment, and isolation.

Emotional Stress and Misunderstandings:

- Fatigue and irritability: The constant fatigue associated with autoimmune diseases can lead to irritability and a short temper. This can strain relationships, as loved ones may misunderstand or become frustrated with the affected individual's behavior.
- Social withdrawal: The physical limitations and emotional toll of autoimmune diseases can make it difficult for individuals to maintain social relationships. This can lead to feelings of loneliness and isolation, further straining family bonds.
- Fear and uncertainty: Living with an autoimmune disease can be a source of fear and uncertainty for both the affected

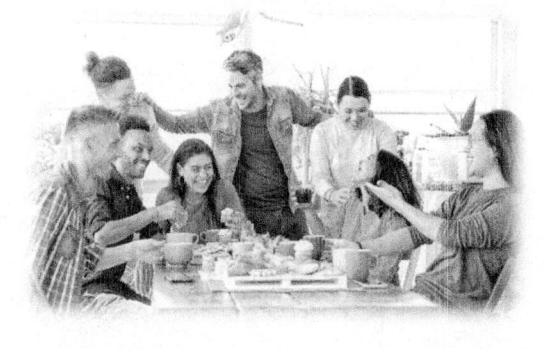

individual and their loved ones. This can create tension and anxiety in relationships.

Caregiver Burden and Stress:
- o Physical and emotional demands: Caregivers of individuals with autoimmune diseases often face significant physical and emotional demands. They may need to assist with daily tasks, provide emotional support, and manage the affected individual's medical appointments.
- o Financial strain: Caring for someone with an autoimmune disease can be financially burdensome, especially if the affected individual is unable to work. This can lead to stress and resentment.
- o Impact on their own lives: Caregivers may sacrifice their own needs and desires to care for their loved ones. This can lead to feelings of burnout and resentment.

Impact on Children:
- o Witnessing parental suffering: Children who witness their parents suffering from an autoimmune disease may experience emotional distress, anxiety, and fear.
- o Changes in family dynamics: The illness can disrupt family routines and dynamics, leading to feelings of insecurity and instability.

- o Need for additional support: Children of parents with autoimmune diseases may require additional emotional and social support.

Economic and Social Consequences

Autoimmune diseases can have significant economic and social consequences for both individuals and families. The high cost of medical care, lost income, and social isolation can create a substantial burden.

Medical Costs:
- o Treatment expenses: The treatment of autoimmune diseases can be expensive, often requiring ongoing medication, therapy, and medical appointments.
- o Out-of-pocket costs: Even with health insurance, individuals with autoimmune diseases may face significant out-of-pocket costs for copays, deductibles, and medications.
- o Long-term care costs: In severe cases, individuals with autoimmune diseases may require long-term care, which can be extremely expensive.

Lost Income:
- o Inability to work: The symptoms of autoimmune diseases can make it difficult or impossible for individuals to work. This can lead to a significant loss of income.

- Disability benefits: Individuals who are unable to work may be eligible for disability benefits, but these benefits are often insufficient to meet their needs.
- Job discrimination: Individuals with autoimmune diseases may face discrimination in the workplace, making it difficult to find and maintain employment.

Social Isolation:
- Limited mobility: The physical limitations of autoimmune diseases can make it difficult for individuals to participate in social activities.
- Stigma and discrimination: Individuals with autoimmune diseases may face stigma and discrimination, leading to social isolation.
- Impact on relationships: The challenges of living with an autoimmune disease can strain relationships with friends and family, leading to feelings of loneliness and isolation.

Impact on Communities:
- Increased healthcare costs: The prevalence of autoimmune diseases can increase healthcare costs for communities and governments.
- Economic burden: The economic consequences of autoimmune diseases can have a negative impact on local economies.

- Need for support services: Communities may need to provide support services for individuals with autoimmune diseases and their families.

Addressing the Economic and Social Consequences:
- ✓ Advocacy: Raising awareness of the economic and social consequences of autoimmune diseases can help to ensure that individuals with these conditions receive the support and resources they need.
- ✓ Access to affordable healthcare: Ensuring access to affordable healthcare is essential for individuals with autoimmune diseases. This may involve expanding health insurance coverage, lowering prescription drug costs, and increasing funding for medical research.
- ✓ Support services: Communities should provide support services for individuals with autoimmune diseases and their families, including counseling, support groups, and educational resources.
- ✓ Workplace accommodations: Employers should make reasonable accommodations for employees with autoimmune diseases, allowing them to continue working and contributing to the workforce.

- ✓ Disability benefits: Governments should ensure that individuals with autoimmune diseases who are unable to work have access to adequate disability benefits.

TRADITIONAL MEDICAL APPROACHES

Medications and Their Side Effects

Traditional medical approaches often involve the use of medications to manage the symptoms of autoimmune diseases. While these medications can be effective in controlling symptoms, they may also have side effects.

Disease-Modifying Anti-Rheumatic Drugs (DMARDs):
- Methotrexate: A commonly used DMARD that can help reduce inflammation and joint damage. However, methotrexate can have side effects such as liver damage, nausea, and hair loss.
- Hydroxychloroquine: A DMARD that can help manage symptoms of autoimmune diseases such as lupus and rheumatoid arthritis. However, hydroxychloroquine can cause vision problems, especially if taken in high doses.

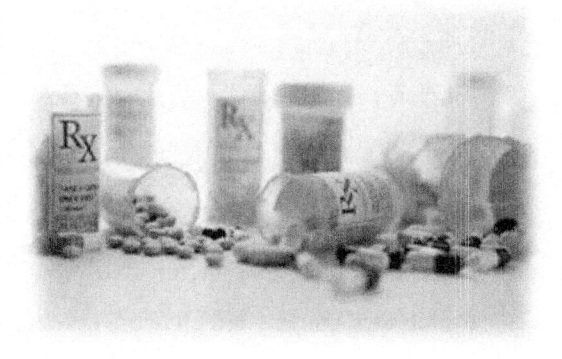

- Sulfasalazine: A DMARD that can help manage symptoms of inflammatory bowel diseases such as ulcerative colitis and Crohn's disease. However, sulfasalazine can cause gastrointestinal side effects such as diarrhea and nausea.

Corticosteroids:
- Prednisone: A powerful anti-inflammatory medication that can help reduce symptoms of autoimmune diseases. However, long-term use of corticosteroids can have side effects such as weight gain, high blood pressure, and osteoporosis.
- Hydrocortisone: A milder corticosteroid that can be used to treat flare-ups of autoimmune diseases. However, hydrocortisone can also cause side effects such as insomnia and increased appetite.

Biologics:
- TNF inhibitors: A class of biologics that target tumor necrosis factor (TNF), a protein involved in inflammation. TNF inhibitors can be effective in treating autoimmune diseases such as rheumatoid arthritis and psoriasis. However, they can also increase the risk of infections.
- Interleukin inhibitors: A class of biologics that target interleukin, another protein involved in inflammation. Interleukin inhibitors can be effective in treating autoimmune

diseases such as Crohn's disease and psoriasis. However, they can also increase the risk of infections.

Other Medications:

- o Nonsteroidal anti-inflammatory drugs (NSAIDs): NSAIDs can help reduce pain and inflammation associated with autoimmune diseases. However, NSAIDs can increase the risk of stomach ulcers and bleeding.
- o Immunosuppressants: Immunosuppressants can help suppress the immune system, reducing inflammation and symptoms of autoimmune diseases. However, immunosuppressants can increase the risk of infections and other serious side effects.

Surgery and Its Risks

Surgery can be a necessary treatment option for some autoimmune diseases. However, surgery carries risks and complications.

Types of Surgery for Autoimmune Diseases:
- o Joint replacement surgery: This may be necessary for individuals with severe joint damage due to autoimmune diseases such as rheumatoid arthritis.

- o Organ transplantation: In some cases, organ transplantation may be necessary to treat autoimmune diseases that affect organs such as the kidneys or liver.
- o Removal of affected tissue: Surgery may be used to remove affected tissue in autoimmune diseases such as Graves' disease or Hashimoto's thyroiditis.

Risks and Complications of Surgery:
- o Infection: Surgery can increase the risk of infection, especially in individuals with weakened immune systems.
- o Bleeding: There is a risk of bleeding during and after surgery.
- o Anesthesia risks: General anesthesia can carry risks, such as nausea, vomiting, and respiratory problems.
- o Complications related to the surgery: The specific risks and complications of surgery will depend on the type of surgery being performed.

It is important to discuss the potential risks and benefits of surgery with your healthcare provider. They can help you weigh the risks and benefits and determine if surgery is the right treatment option for you.

The Limitations of Conventional Treatments

While traditional medical approaches can be effective in managing the symptoms of autoimmune diseases, they have limitations.

- Symptom management: Many conventional treatments focus on managing the symptoms of autoimmune diseases rather than addressing the underlying cause.
- Side effects: Many medications used to treat autoimmune diseases have side effects that can be serious and debilitating.
- Limited effectiveness: In some cases, conventional treatments may not be effective in controlling the symptoms of autoimmune diseases.
- High cost: The cost of treating autoimmune diseases can be high, especially for individuals who require ongoing medication or therapy.

THE SEARCH FOR CURES

Current Research and Advancements

The field of autoimmune disease research is constantly evolving, with new discoveries and advancements being made every year. Scientists are working to better understand the underlying causes of these complex conditions and develop more effective treatments.

Immunotherapy:

One promising area of research is immunotherapy, which aims to modulate the immune system to reduce inflammation and prevent tissue damage. This approach includes:

- Biological agents: These are drugs that target specific molecules involved in the immune system, such as tumor necrosis factor (TNF) and interleukin-1 (IL-1). Examples of biological agents include adalimumab, infliximab, and etanercept.

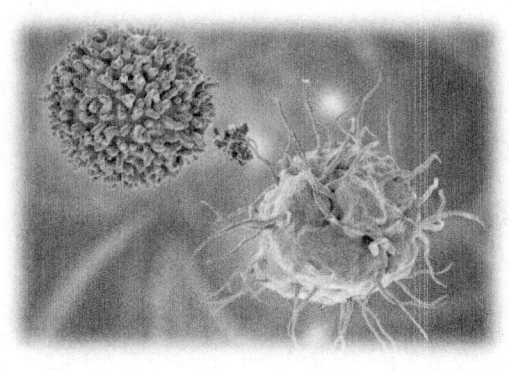

- Cell therapy: This involves using a patient's own immune cells or engineered cells to treat autoimmune diseases. For example, chimeric antigen receptor (CAR) T cell therapy has shown promise in treating certain types of autoimmune diseases.

Gene therapy:
Gene therapy aims to correct genetic defects that contribute to autoimmune diseases. This involves introducing healthy genes into cells to replace faulty ones. While still in the experimental stages, gene therapy has shown potential in treating certain inherited autoimmune diseases.

Nanotechnology:
Nanotechnology involves using tiny particles to deliver drugs or other treatments to specific cells or tissues. This approach has the potential to improve the efficacy of treatments while reducing side effects.

Stem cell therapy:
Stem cell therapy involves using stem cells to regenerate damaged tissues and organs. This approach has shown promise in treating autoimmune diseases such as multiple sclerosis and type 1 diabetes.

Precision medicine:
Precision medicine involves tailoring treatments to the individual needs of each patient based on their genetic makeup and other factors. This

approach has the potential to improve treatment outcomes and reduce side effects.

Emerging Therapies and Their Potential

In addition to the current research and advancements, several emerging therapies show promise in the treatment of autoimmune diseases.

Gut microbiome modulation:

The gut microbiome plays a crucial role in immune function. Research suggests that modulating the gut microbiome may be beneficial in treating autoimmune diseases. This can be achieved through dietary changes, probiotics, or fecal microbiota transplantation.

Metabolic therapies:

Some autoimmune diseases are associated with metabolic abnormalities. Targeting these abnormalities may be beneficial in treating the underlying disease. For example, dietary changes and medications that improve glucose control may be helpful in managing autoimmune diseases such as type 1 diabetes and rheumatoid arthritis.

Artificial intelligence (AI):

AI can be used to analyze large datasets of patient information and identify patterns that may be relevant to autoimmune diseases. This can help researchers develop new treatments and improve patient care.

Organoids:

Organoids are three-dimensional cell cultures that mimic the structure and function of organs. These can be used to study autoimmune diseases and develop new treatments.

The Challenges in Developing Effective Treatments

Despite significant advancements in research, developing effective treatments for autoimmune diseases remains a complex and challenging task. Several factors contribute to these challenges:

1. Heterogeneity of Autoimmune Diseases:

- Diverse manifestations: Autoimmune diseases are a heterogeneous group of conditions with varying symptoms and severity. This makes it difficult to develop treatments that are effective for all patients.
- Disease subtypes: Many autoimmune diseases have different subtypes, each with its own unique characteristics and treatment requirements.

2. Complexity of the Immune System:

- Understanding the underlying mechanisms: The immune system is a complex network of cells and molecules that interact in intricate ways. Understanding the specific mechanisms involved in autoimmune diseases is essential for developing targeted treatments.
- Balancing immune responses: Autoimmune diseases involve an overactive immune system. Treatments must strike a delicate balance between suppressing the immune system to reduce inflammation and maintaining a healthy immune response to protect against infections.

3. Limited Understanding of Etiology:

- Unknown causes: The exact causes of many autoimmune diseases remain unknown, making it difficult to develop targeted treatments.
- Environmental factors: Environmental factors, such as infections, toxins, and stress, may play a role in triggering autoimmune diseases. Identifying these factors can be challenging.

4. Clinical Trial Challenges:

- Recruitment difficulties: Recruiting patients for clinical trials of autoimmune diseases can be difficult due to the rarity of

some conditions and the challenges of enrolling individuals with diverse symptoms and backgrounds.
- Long-term follow-up: Evaluating the effectiveness and safety of treatments for autoimmune diseases often requires long-term follow-up, which can be challenging and expensive.

5. Regulatory Hurdles:

- Complex approval process: The process of obtaining regulatory approval for new treatments can be lengthy and complex.
- Cost and access: Even after approval, new treatments may be expensive and difficult to access for patients.

LIFESTYLE AND ENVIRONMENTAL FACTORS

The Role of Diet and Nutrition

Diet and nutrition play a crucial role in managing autoimmune diseases. While there is no one-size-fits-all diet for autoimmune diseases, some dietary changes may be beneficial.

Anti-inflammatory Diet:
- Foods to include: Fruits, vegetables, whole grains, lean proteins, and healthy fats.
- Foods to limit: Processed foods, sugary drinks, red meat, and refined carbohydrates.
- Supplements: Some people with autoimmune diseases may benefit from taking supplements such as omega-3 fatty acids, vitamin D, and probiotics.

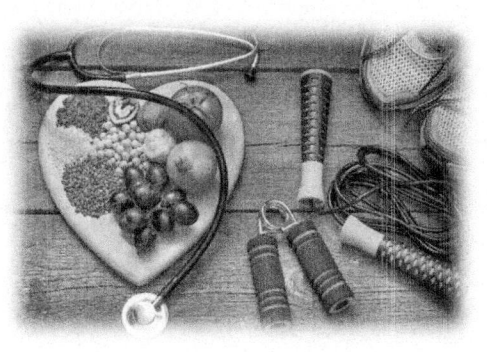

Elimination Diets:
- Identifying triggers: Elimination diets involve eliminating certain foods from the diet to see if they trigger symptoms.

Common foods that may be eliminated include gluten, dairy, and nightshades.
- Reintroduction: After a period of elimination, foods are gradually reintroduced to identify any triggers.

Personalized Nutrition:
- o Working with a registered dietitian: A registered dietitian can help individuals with autoimmune diseases develop a personalized nutrition plan that meets their specific needs.

Important Considerations:
- o Individual variations: The best diet for an individual with an autoimmune disease may vary depending on the specific condition, symptoms, and personal preferences.
- o Consulting with a healthcare provider: It is important to consult with a healthcare provider before making any significant changes to your diet.

Stress Management and Relaxation Techniques

Stress can exacerbate the symptoms of autoimmune diseases. Effective stress management techniques can help reduce stress and improve overall well-being.

Stress Management Techniques:
- o Mindfulness and meditation: Mindfulness and meditation can help reduce stress and improve focus.
- o Deep breathing exercises: Deep breathing exercises can help calm the mind and body.
- o Yoga and tai chi: These practices can improve flexibility, strength, and balance, while also reducing stress.

- Spending time in nature: Spending time in nature can have a calming and restorative effect.
- Social support: Connecting with friends and family can provide emotional support and reduce stress.

Finding What Works for You:
- Experimentation: It may take some experimentation to find the stress management techniques that work best for you.
- Seeking professional help: If you are struggling to manage stress, consider seeking professional help from a therapist or counselor.

Exercise and Physical Activity

Regular exercise can have numerous benefits for individuals with autoimmune diseases. It can help improve physical function, reduce pain, and boost mood.

Benefits of Exercise:
- Improved physical function: Exercise can help improve muscle strength, flexibility, and endurance.
- Reduced pain: Regular physical activity can help reduce joint pain and stiffness.
- Boosted mood: Exercise can help improve mood and reduce stress.
- Weight management: Maintaining a healthy weight can help manage the symptoms of some autoimmune diseases.

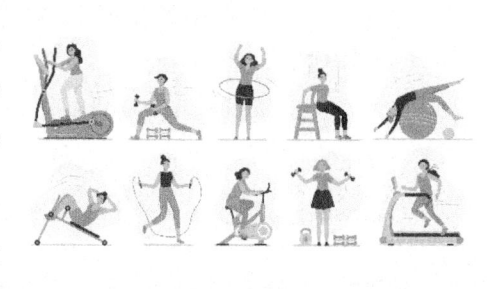

Types of Exercise:
- Low-impact exercises: Activities such as swimming, cycling, and yoga are gentle on the joints and can be beneficial for individuals with autoimmune diseases.
- Strength training: Building muscle can help improve physical function and reduce pain.

- o Flexibility exercises: Stretching can help improve range of motion and reduce stiffness.

Important Considerations:
- Listening to your body: It is important to listen to your body and avoid overexertion.
- Consulting with a healthcare provider: Before starting an exercise program, it is important to consult with a healthcare provider to ensure it is safe for you.

Environmental Toxins and Their Impact

Exposure to environmental toxins can trigger or exacerbate the symptoms of autoimmune diseases. Identifying and avoiding these toxins can be important for managing the condition.

Common Environmental Toxins:
- Air pollution: Exposure to air pollution can trigger or worsen symptoms of autoimmune diseases such as asthma and lupus.
- Chemical exposure: Exposure to chemicals found in household products, pesticides, and other sources can also trigger or worsen symptoms.

- Electromagnetic fields: Exposure to electromagnetic fields (EMFs) from electronic devices and power lines may contribute to autoimmune diseases.
- Reducing Exposure to Environmental Toxins:

- Air quality: Use air purifiers and avoid outdoor activities on days with poor air quality.
- Chemical exposure: Choose natural cleaning products and avoid exposure to pesticides and other chemicals.
- EMF exposure: Limit your use of electronic devices and avoid sleeping near electrical outlets or power lines.

Important Considerations:

- Individual sensitivity: People may have different sensitivities to environmental toxins.
- Consulting with a healthcare provider: If you suspect that environmental toxins are contributing to your autoimmune disease symptoms, consult with a healthcare provider.

ACUPUNCTURE AND ACUPRESSURE

Acupuncture and Acupressure

Acupuncture and acupressure are traditional Chinese medicine practices that involve stimulating specific points on the body.

Acupuncture:

- Thin needles: Acupuncture involves inserting thin needles into specific points on the body.
- Meridians: These points are believed to be connected by energy pathways called meridians.
- Balancing energy flow: Acupuncture is believed to balance the flow of energy (qi) through the body, promoting healing and well-being.

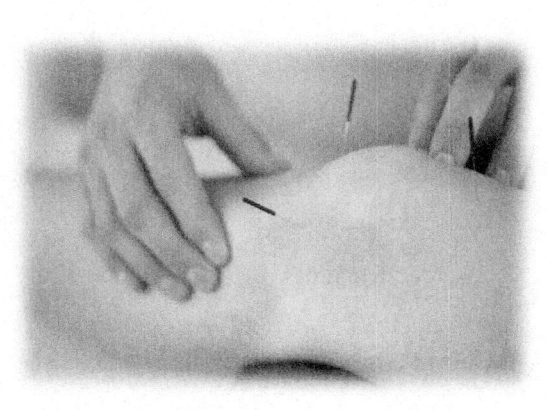

Acupressure:

- Finger pressure: Acupressure involves applying pressure to specific points on the body with your fingers.

- Similar benefits: Acupressure is believed to have similar benefits to acupuncture.

Potential Benefits:
- Pain relief: Acupuncture and acupressure may be effective in reducing pain associated with autoimmune diseases.
- Improved immune function: Some studies suggest that acupuncture and acupressure may help boost the immune system.
- Reduced stress: Acupuncture and acupressure may help reduce stress and anxiety.

Important Considerations:
- Qualified practitioner: It is important to seek treatment from a qualified practitioner who is trained in acupuncture or acupressure.
- Potential side effects: Acupuncture and acupressure are generally safe, but there may be some risks such as bruising or infection.
- Herbal Remedies and Supplements
- Herbal remedies and supplements are natural products that may be used to treat autoimmune diseases.

Common Herbal Remedies:
- Turmeric: Turmeric contains curcumin, a compound with anti-inflammatory properties.
- Ginger: Ginger has anti-inflammatory and antioxidant properties.
- Boswellia: Boswellia is a resin derived from the Boswellia serrata tree and has anti-inflammatory properties.
- Ashwagandha: Ashwagandha is an adaptogen that can help reduce stress and improve immune function.

Potential Benefits:
- Reduced inflammation: Some herbal remedies may help reduce inflammation associated with autoimmune diseases.
- Improved immune function: Certain herbs may help boost the immune system.
- Reduced stress: Some herbs can help reduce stress and anxiety.

Important Considerations:
- Quality and purity: It is important to ensure that herbal remedies and supplements are of high quality and purity.
- Potential interactions: Herbal remedies and supplements may interact with medications or other herbs.

Chiropractic Care and Massage Therapy

Chiropractic care and massage therapy are two complementary and alternative medicine (CAM) therapies that may be beneficial for individuals with autoimmune diseases.

Chiropractic Care:
- o Spinal manipulation: Chiropractic care involves manipulating the spine to improve alignment and reduce pain.
- o Nervous system function: Chiropractors believe that spinal misalignment can interfere with the nervous system and contribute to health problems.
- o Potential benefits: Chiropractic care may help reduce pain, improve mobility, and boost the immune system.

Massage Therapy:
- o Manual manipulation: Massage therapy involves the manipulation of soft tissues to relieve pain and tension.
- o Relaxation and stress reduction: Massage therapy can help promote relaxation and reduce stress.
- o Improved circulation: Massage therapy can help improve blood flow and circulation.

Potential Benefits of Chiropractic Care and Massage Therapy:
- Pain relief: Both chiropractic care and massage therapy may be effective in reducing pain associated with autoimmune diseases.
- Improved mobility: Chiropractic care and massage therapy can help improve range of motion and flexibility.
- Reduced stress: These therapies can help reduce stress and anxiety, which can be beneficial for individuals with autoimmune diseases.

Important Considerations:
- Qualified practitioner: It is important to seek treatment from a qualified chiropractor or massage therapist.
- Potential side effects: While chiropractic care and massage therapy are generally safe, there may be some risks such as bruising or discomfort.
- Combining with other treatments: These therapies may be most effective when combined with other treatments, such as conventional medical care.

Mindfulness and Meditation

Mindfulness and meditation are mind-body practices that can help reduce stress and improve overall well-being.

Mindfulness:
- Present-moment awareness: Mindfulness involves paying attention to the present moment without judgment.
- Reduced stress: Mindfulness can help reduce stress and anxiety.
- Improved focus: Mindfulness can help improve focus and concentration.

Meditation:
- Relaxation techniques: Meditation involves various relaxation techniques, such as deep breathing and visualization.
- Reduced stress and anxiety: Meditation can help reduce stress and anxiety.

Improved sleep: Meditation may also help improve sleep quality.

Potential Benefits of Mindfulness and Meditation:
- Reduced stress and anxiety: Mindfulness and meditation can help reduce stress and anxiety, which can be beneficial for individuals with autoimmune diseases.
- Improved mood: These practices can help improve mood and overall well-being.

- o Enhanced immune function: Some studies suggest that mindfulness and meditation may help boost the immune system.

Important Considerations:
- o Guided meditation: Guided meditation can be helpful for beginners.
- o Regular practice: Mindfulness and meditation are most effective when practiced regularly.

HOLISTIC APPROACHES TO HEALING

The Mind-Body Connection

The mind-body connection refers to the idea that the mind and body are interconnected and influence each other. This concept is central to many holistic approaches to healing.

The Role of Stress and Emotions:

- o Stress and inflammation: Chronic stress can contribute to inflammation, which is a key factor in many autoimmune diseases.
- o Emotional well-being: Emotional factors such as anxiety, depression, and trauma can also impact the immune system and contribute to the development of autoimmune diseases.

The Importance of Positive Emotions:

- o Healing and resilience: Positive emotions such as gratitude, joy, and compassion can promote healing and resilience.

- Immune function: Research suggests that positive emotions can boost the immune system and improve overall health.

Mindfulness and Meditation:
- Stress reduction: Mindfulness and meditation can help reduce stress and promote relaxation.
- Improved immune function: These practices may also help improve immune function and reduce inflammation.

Emotional and Spiritual Well-Being

Emotional and spiritual well-being are essential components of holistic healing.

Addressing Emotional Issues:
- Therapy: Psychotherapy can help individuals with autoimmune diseases address emotional issues such as anxiety, depression, and trauma.
- Support groups: Connecting with others who have autoimmune diseases can provide emotional support and a sense of community.

Exploring Spirituality:
- Finding meaning: Exploring spirituality can help individuals find meaning and purpose in their lives, even in the face of challenges.

- Connection to something larger: A spiritual connection can provide a sense of peace and comfort.

Holistic Healing Practices:
- Yoga and tai chi: These practices can help improve physical and emotional well-being.
- Qi gong: Qi gong is a Chinese practice that involves movement, breathing, and meditation.
- Art therapy: Art therapy can be a powerful tool for expressing emotions and promoting healing.

Important Considerations:
- Individualized approach: The best holistic healing practices will vary from person to person.
- Complementary to conventional medicine: Holistic approaches should be used in conjunction with conventional medical care.
- Seeking professional guidance: It is important to seek guidance from qualified professionals who specialize in holistic healing.

Personalized Healing Plans

Holistic healing plans should be tailored to the individual needs and preferences of each person. It is important to work with a qualified healthcare provider or holistic practitioner to develop a personalized plan.

Key Components of a Personalized Healing Plan:
- **Assessment of individual needs:** A comprehensive assessment should be conducted to identify the individual's physical, emotional, and spiritual needs.
- **Goal setting:** Clear and achievable goals should be set to guide the healing process.
- **Treatment plan:** A personalized treatment plan should be developed based on the individual's needs and preferences.
- **Monitoring and evaluation:** The effectiveness of the treatment plan should be monitored and evaluated regularly.

Examples of Personalized Healing Plans:
- **Mind-body medicine:** A personalized healing plan may include mind-body practices such as mindfulness, meditation, yoga, or tai chi.
- **Nutritional therapy:** A registered dietitian can help develop a personalized nutrition plan that addresses the individual's specific needs.

- **Herbal remedies and supplements:** Carefully selected herbal remedies and supplements may be incorporated into a personalized healing plan.
- **Complementary therapies:** Other complementary therapies, such as acupuncture, massage therapy, or chiropractic care, may also be included in the plan.

Important Considerations:
- **Individual variation:** The best healing plan will vary from person to person.
- **Collaboration with healthcare providers:** It is important to collaborate with healthcare providers to ensure that a personalized healing plan is safe and effective.
- **Patience and persistence:** Healing can take time, and it is important to be patient and persistent.

PERSONAL NARRATIVES

Inspiring Stories of Individuals Overcoming Autoimmune Challenges

The following are inspiring real life stories of individuals who have overcome the challenges of living with autoimmune diseases.

Story 1: Maria's Journey with Lupus

Maria was diagnosed with lupus at a young age. The fatigue, joint pain, and skin rashes were debilitating, and she often felt isolated and alone. However, Maria refused to let lupus define her. She joined a support group, learned about her condition, and made lifestyle changes to manage her symptoms. With the support of her family and friends, Maria was able to overcome the challenges of lupus and live a fulfilling life.

Story 2: David's Triumph Over Multiple Sclerosis

David was diagnosed with multiple sclerosis (MS) in his early 30s. The physical and emotional challenges of MS were overwhelming, but David was determined to maintain a positive outlook. He embraced a healthy lifestyle, joined a support group, and explored alternative therapies. With the support of his loved ones, David was able to overcome the limitations of MS and live a full and active life.

Story 3: Sarah's Resilience with Crohn's Disease

Sarah was diagnosed with Crohn's disease as a teenager. The constant pain, fatigue, and digestive problems were debilitating, but Sarah refused to let Crohn's control her life. She learned about her condition, made dietary changes, and sought medical treatment. With the support of her family and friends, Sarah was able to manage her symptoms and pursue her dreams.

Story 4: Michael's Hope in the Face of Rheumatoid Arthritis

Michael was diagnosed with rheumatoid arthritis in his 40s. The joint pain and stiffness were so severe that he could barely walk. However, Michael refused to give up. He sought medical treatment, joined a support group, and made lifestyle changes. With the support of his loved ones, Michael was able to manage his symptoms and live a fulfilling life.

Story 5: Emily's Triumph Over Type 1 Diabetes

Emily was diagnosed with type 1 diabetes as a child. The daily insulin injections, blood sugar monitoring, and dietary restrictions were challenging, but Emily was determined to live a normal life. She learned about her condition, developed a healthy lifestyle, and joined a support group. With the support of her family and friends, Emily was able to manage her diabetes and achieve her goals.

These are just a few examples of individuals who have overcome the challenges of living with autoimmune diseases. Their stories can be a source of inspiration and hope for others who are facing similar challenges.

Lessons Learned and Strategies for Coping

The individuals in these stories have learned valuable lessons about living with autoimmune diseases and have developed strategies for coping with the challenges.

Lessons Learned:

- **The importance of support:** Having a strong support system is crucial for individuals with autoimmune diseases.
- **The power of positivity:** A positive outlook can help individuals cope with the challenges of living with an autoimmune disease.
- **The value of knowledge:** Learning about the condition and its management can empower individuals to take control of their health.
- **The importance of self-care:** Taking care of oneself physically, emotionally, and spiritually is essential for managing autoimmune diseases.

- **The power of resilience:** Resilience is key to overcoming the challenges of living with an autoimmune disease.

Strategies for Coping:
- **Seeking support:** Connecting with others who have autoimmune diseases can provide emotional support and a sense of community.
- **Practicing self-care:** Engaging in activities that promote physical, emotional, and spiritual well-being.
- **Developing a support system:** Building a strong network of friends and family who can provide support and encouragement.
- **Learning about the condition:** Educating oneself about the autoimmune disease and its management can help individuals make informed decisions about their healthcare.
- **Setting realistic goals:** Setting achievable goals can help individuals maintain a sense of purpose and accomplishment.
- **Finding meaning:** Exploring spirituality or other meaningful activities can help individuals find purpose and meaning in their lives.

HOPE FOR THE FUTURE

The Power of Advocacy and Awareness

Advocacy and awareness are essential for advancing research, improving access to care, and reducing the stigma associated with autoimmune diseases.

Advocacy:
- o Government lobbying: Advocating for government policies that support research, funding, and patient rights can help improve the lives of individuals with autoimmune diseases.
- o Community engagement: Engaging with the community can help raise awareness of autoimmune diseases and reduce stigma.
- o Support groups: Joining or forming support groups can provide a platform for advocacy and networking.

Awareness:
- o Education and information: Educating the public about autoimmune diseases can help reduce stigma and promote understanding.
- o Media campaigns: Media campaigns can raise awareness of autoimmune diseases and the challenges faced by individuals with these conditions.

- Social media: Using social media to share personal stories and information about autoimmune diseases can help raise awareness and connect with others.

Embracing a Positive Outlook

A positive outlook can be a powerful tool for coping with the challenges of living with an autoimmune disease.

Benefits of a Positive Outlook:
- Improved mental health: A positive outlook can help reduce stress, anxiety, and depression.
- Enhanced immune function: Research suggests that a positive outlook can boost the immune system.
- Increased resilience: A positive outlook can help individuals develop resilience and cope with challenges more effectively.

Strategies for Embracing a Positive Outlook:
- Gratitude practice: Focusing on the positive aspects of life can help cultivate a positive outlook.
- Mindfulness and meditation: These practices can help reduce stress and promote a positive mindset.
- Surrounding yourself with positivity: Spending time with positive and supportive people can help uplift your spirits.
- Setting goals: Setting achievable goals can provide a sense of purpose and motivation.

- o   Finding meaning: Exploring spirituality or other meaningful activities can help individuals find purpose and hope.

The Potential for a Brighter Future

Despite the challenges posed by autoimmune diseases, there is hope for a brighter future. Advancements in research, improved access to care, and increased awareness are all contributing to a more positive outlook.

Research and Development:
- o   Continued advancements: Research into autoimmune diseases is ongoing, with the potential for significant breakthroughs in the years to come.
- o   New treatments and therapies: Emerging therapies such as gene therapy, stem cell therapy, and precision medicine hold promise for improving treatment outcomes.
- o   Personalized medicine: The development of personalized treatment plans based on individual genetic makeup and other factors can help optimize care.

Improved Access to Care:
- o Expanded healthcare coverage: Efforts to expand healthcare coverage can help ensure that individuals with autoimmune diseases have access to the care they need.
- o Reduced healthcare disparities: Addressing healthcare disparities can help ensure that everyone has equal access to quality care, regardless of their socioeconomic status or geographic location.

Increased Awareness and Support:
- o Community engagement: Raising awareness of autoimmune diseases and the challenges faced by individuals with these conditions can help reduce stigma and promote understanding.
- o Support networks: Building strong support networks can provide individuals with emotional support, information, and resources.

Embracing Hope:
- o Positive outlook: Maintaining a positive outlook can help individuals with autoimmune diseases cope with challenges and find meaning in their lives.
- o Resilience: Developing resilience can help individuals overcome obstacles and persevere in the face of adversity.

PERSONAL NOTES

Printed in Great Britain
by Amazon